CONTENTS

Introduction

Inflammation is a normal procedure that enables your body to recuperate and guard itself against hurt. Nonetheless, inflammation is destructive if it gets chronic. Chronic inflammation may keep going for quite a long time, months, or years and may prompt different medical issues. So, there are numerous things you can do to diminish inflammation and improve your general wellbeing. This article diagrams a point by point plan for an anti-inflammatory diet and way of life.

Be that as it may, once in a while inflammation continues, all day every day, in any event, when an outside intruder does not compromise you. That is when inflammation can turn into your foe. Many significant sicknesses that plague us, including malignant growth, coronary illness, diabetes, joint pain, sorrow, and Alzheimer's have been connected to chronic inflammation.

One of the most incredible assets to battle inflammation comes not from the drug store, yet the market. "Numerous exploratory examinations have indicated that segments of nourishments or drinks may have anti-inflammatory impacts," says Dr Candid Hu, teacher of sustenance and the study of disease transmission in the Department of Nutrition at the Harvard School of Public Health.

Nourishments that cause inflammation

Attempt to keep away from or limit these nourishments however much as could reasonably be expected:

- refined starches, for example, white bread and baked goods
- French fries and other seared nourishments
- pop and other sugar-improved drinks
- red meat (burgers, steaks) and handled meat (sausages, hotdog)
- margarine, shortening, and fat

Anti-Inflammatory Diet Recipes

Followings are 20+ anti-inflammatory diet recipes you should try now.

1.Oat porridge with berries

- Cook time: 30 mins
- Absolute time: 30 mins

INGREDIENTS

For the oats:

- 1 cup steel-cut oats (search for guaranteed without gluten on the off chance that you have a gluten intolerance)
- 3 cups of water
- touch of salt
- For fixing (these are for the most part discretionary, and to-taste):
- new or solidified natural product/berries (I utilized blueberries and raspberries, yet any organic product will work)
- a bunch of cut almonds, pepitas, hemp seeds, or another nut/seed (you could even utilize a tad bit of your preferred granola - I'm an enthusiast of this Honey and Hazelnut Granola)
- unsweetened kefir, handcrafted or locally acquired
- shower of maple syrup, a sprinkling of coconut sugar, a couple of drops of stevia, or some other sugar you like, to taste

Directions

Add the oats to a little pot and spot over medium-high warmth. Permit to toast, mixing or shaking the skillet as often as possible, for 2-3 minutes.

Add the water and heat to the point of boiling. Diminish the warmth to a stew, and let cook for around 25 minutes, or until the oats are delicate enough for your enjoying. (The oats will thicken up as they cool - on the off chance that you lean toward them more porridgy, include a sprinkle more water, or some milk or without dairy elective.)

Present with berries, nuts/seeds (or a bunch of granola), a sprinkle of kefir, and any sugar you like, to taste. Delve in!

NOTES

This makes enough oats for around four servings; however, I prefer to twofold this and have cooked oats in the ice chest for simple weekday morning meals for the spouse and myself. Remaining oats can be warmed in the microwave (if they've gotten somewhat thick, include a sprinkle of water, milk, or sans dairy substitute) and you're ready! P.S., my companion Aysegul simply shared a post on her blog about making steel cut oats in a moderate cooker. She has a virtuoso method that permits you to get the oats cooking before bed, and afterwards wake up to warm, superbly creamy porridge toward the beginning of the day.

2.Buckwheat and chia seed porridge

- Cook time: 20min

INGREDIENTS

- 1 cup buckwheat, flushed
- ½ cup oats
- Two tablespoons chia seeds
- 2 cups milk (cow's, almond or soy)
- 2 cups of water
- One every pear and apple, ground with skin on
- One teaspoon each ground ginger and cinnamon
- ½ teaspoon each ground nutmeg and cardamom
- Two tablespoons nut margarine
- One teaspoon vanilla concentrate
- Two tablespoons nectar
- Blended Berry Compote
- 500 grams blended solidified berries
- finely ground pizzazz and juice one orange
- ⅓ cup caster sugar
- Two teaspoons cornflour
- One tablespoon water

Directions

Put the buckwheat and oats in a bowl and spread well with cold water. Put the chia seeds in a different bowl and include 1 cup of the milk. Leave the two dishes on the seat to douse medium-term.

Channel the buckwheat and oats in a fine strainer at that point wash thoroughly under virus water.

Spot the chia seeds with the milk in a medium pot alongside the staying 1 cup milk, the buckwheat and oats, water, ground pear and apple, all the flavours, nut spread, vanilla and nectar. Cook over low warmth for around 30 minutes, frequently blending until thick and velvety, adding more water or milk to keep it at a delicate consistency. Serve in bowls bested with your selection of INGREDIENTS.

Cook's tip: The porridge keeps well in the cooler for five days. Simply heat each serving when required, including some additional fluid if necessary.

Blended Berry Compote

Put the berries, orange get-up-and-go and squeeze and the caster sugar in a pot and gradually bring to the bubble. Combine the corn flour and water in a bowl until smooth at that point mix into the berries. Stew for a few minutes until the juices have thickened. Serve warm or at room temperature. Makes around 2 cups

Beating recommendations

Milk or cream or a non-dairy milk, for example, almond or soy; coconut yoghurt or ordinary yoghurt – plain or organic product; simmered figs with nectar; new berries when in season; cinnamon-broiled pears or apples; poached rhubarb with raspberries; cut banana and maple syrup; toasted nuts and seeds – almonds, macadamias, walnuts, pecans, hazelnuts, pistachios, sesame, sunflower and pumpkin seeds.

3.Fried eggs with turmeric

- cook time: 45min

INGREDIENTS

- 3 unfenced or natural eggs
- One teaspoon new ground turmeric (see notes)
- One teaspoon chia seeds
- Two tablespoons natural coconut milk or cream
- Squeeze ocean salt
- Two teaspoons cold squeezed olive oil
- 100 g infant spinach leaves
- One tablespoon Super Greens Pesto (see beneath)

Directions

Whisk eggs, chia turmeric, ocean salt and coconut milk in a bowl until joined, at that point put in a safe spot.

Pour one teaspoon of the olive oil into a skillet over a low to medium warmth.

Include the spinach and sauté delicately for 30 seconds until shrivelled.

Expel spinach from the warmth.

Warmth a little 20 cm skillet over medium heat with one teaspoon olive oil.

Pour in the egg blend and delicately mix through until the eggs begin to set and get rich.

Include the wilted spinach and crease through.

Serve quickly in the container with Super Greens Pesto and appreciate.

4. Smoked salmon, avocado, and poached eggs on toast

- Planning Time 10 minutes
- Cook Time 4 minutes

INGREDIENTS

With soy sauce and sesame seeds.

- Two cuts of bread toasted
- 1/2 enormous avocado crushed
- 1/4 tsp crisply crushed lemon juice
- Spot of fit salt and broke dark pepper
- 3.5 oz smoked salmon

- Two eggs, poached *see notes
- Sprinkle of Kikkoman soy sauce discretionary
- 1 TBSP meagerly cut scallions
- Microgreens discretionary

With tomato and everything bagel flavouring.

- Two cuts of bread
- 1/2 enormous avocado
- 1/4 tsp crisply crushed lemon juice
- Touch of genuine salt and split dark pepper
- 3.5 oz smoked salmon

- Two eggs, poached *See notes
- Two slender cuts of tomato
- 1 tsp Everything Bagel Seasoning
- Microgreens

Directions

In a little bowl, crush the avocado. Include the lemon juice and a touch of salt; blend well and put in a safe spot.

Poach your eggs (see notes) and, when they are sitting in the ice shower, toast your bread.

When your bread is toasted, spread the avocado on the two cuts and add the smoked salmon to each cut.

Cautiously move the poached eggs to their separate toasts.

Hit with a sprinkle of Kikkoman soy sauce and some broke pepper; embellish with scallions and microgreens.

Or on the other hand

Spot cut of tomato on each toast, at that point, hit the toasts with some everything bagel flavouring. Trimming with microgreens.

Notes

! The most effective method to poach an egg: Note: You'll need to steal your eggs individually. Bring a little pot of water to a relentless stew. (A few people include a light sprinkle of vinegar to the sea; I've attempted with and without, and I've never seen an alternate, so I skip it.) Crack your eggs into single ramekins or little bowls. With a spatula or large spoon, make a delicate whirlpool in the stewing water; this will enable the egg to white fold over the yolk. Gently tip the egg into the water whirlpool, white first. Cook for two minutes. Carefully evacuate the egg with an opened spoon. Carefully move the egg to an ice shower for approx. Ten seconds to prevent it from cooking (protein will keep on cooking after it's expelled from heat, so you need to guarantee you get that runny satiny yoke).After a quick dunk into the ice shower, move your egg to a paper towel and delicately pat it dry. Evacuate any wispy white egg with the edge of your spoon, and transfer to your plate.

5.Pineapple smoothie

- planning time: 20min

A heavenly and velvety green kale pineapple smoothie with banana and Greek yoghurt. Loaded up with stable protein, supplements, and will keep you full for a considerable length of time!

INGREDIENTS

- 2 cups softly pressed cleaved kale leaves stems expelled
- 3/4 cup unsweetened vanilla almond milk or any milk you like
- One solidified medium banana cut into lumps
- 1/4 cup plain non-fat Greek yoghurt
- 1/4 cup hardened pineapple pieces
- Two tablespoons nutty spread velvety or crunchy (I utilize characteristic-rich)
- 1 to 3 teaspoons nectar to taste

Guidelines

Spot all INGREDIENTS (kale, almond milk, banana, yoghurt, pineapple, nutty spread, and nectar) in a blender in the request recorded. Mix until smooth. Add more milk varying to arrive at the desired consistency. Appreciate right away.

6.Barbecued sauerkraut, hummus, and avocado sandwich

- Cook Time: 12 mins
- Absolute Time: 22 mins

INGREDIENTS

- 8 cuts pumpernickel bread
- veggie lover lavish spread (or customary margarine)
- 1 cup hummus (broiled garlic enhance, partitioned)
- 1 cup sauerkraut (depleted, daintily flushed, and fluid crushed out)
- One avocado (stripped and cut the long way into around 16 pieces (you can forget about this fixing on the off chance that you need to bring down the fat substance of the sandwich, and it will, in any case, be extremely delightful!))

Directions

Preheat stove to 450 degrees F (230 degrees C).

Spread margarine on one side of every one of the eight cuts of bread and spotted 4 of them spread side down on a heating sheet.

Take about a portion of the hummus and disseminate over the four cuts of bread.

Disseminate the sauerkraut over the hummus on each cut.

Disseminate the avocado cuts over the sauerkraut.

For the staying four cuts of bread, spread hummus as an afterthought without margarine and spot hummus side down on the avocado cuts.

Prepare in the broiler for 6-8 minutes, at that point, flip the sandwiches and heat around 6 minutes more, until the sandwiches are brilliant dark coloured and firm. (On the other hand, you can flame broil them on the stovetop on a frying pan or in a skillet).

7.Spinach and feta frittata

- cook time: 25min

INGREDIENTS

- 1 tsp olive oil
- ½ little darker onion stripped and finely cut
- 1 tsp garlic
- 250 g infant spinach
- Four eggs
- ½ cup disintegrated feta cheddar
- Salt and pepper to taste
- Spinach and Feta Frittata

Guidelines

Preheat your barbecue to medium-high warmth.

Utilizing a nonstick skillet that you can put under the barbecue, heat the oil over medium warmth.

Include the onion and cook until only beginning to darker. Include the spinach and hurl for a moment or two until it starts to wither. Expel from the warmth and permit to cool.

Beat the eggs in a bowl. Include the cooled spinach and onion, and afterwards the feta — season to taste.

Put your skillet back on a medium warmth and include the eggs. Mix delicately with a spatula until you feel the egg begin to set on the base. Mood killer the heat, so the frittata remains very runny.

Spot your skillet under the flame broil for 2 to 3 minutes, or until the frittata is brilliant and entirely cooked through (check with a fork.)

Spot a plate over the container and turn over rapidly however cautiously to discharge the frittata. Serve hot or cold with a rigid side plate of mixed greens.

8.Quinoa and citrus serving of mixed greens

- Cook time: 20min

INGREDIENTS

- 1 cup cooked quinoa, cooled
- Two little oranges, supreme
- One celery rib, finely slashed
- 20 g Brazil nuts, slashed
- One green onion, cut
- ¼ cup crisp parsley, finely hacked

For the dressing

- juice from above oranges
- ½ tsp lemon juice
- ½ tsp fresh ginger, ground
- 1 tsp white wine vinegar
- One little clove garlic, minced
- ½ tsp salt
- ¼ tsp dark pepper
- squeeze cinnamon

Guidelines

Cut the oranges into supremes, working over a bowl, altogether not lose any of the juice. At the point when you have all your supremes done, make a point to press all the juice out of the "layers" that are deserted.

Move that juice to your small-scale blender or nourishment processor. Include the remainder of the elements for the dressing and mix until smooth.

Cut your orange supremes into reduced down pieces and add them to a medium-size blending bowl. Include the remainder of the INGREDIENTS, including the dressing, and mix until all-around joined.

Serve quickly, or keep in the cooler until prepared to serve.

NOTES

Gluten-Free, Grain-Free

9.Lentil, beetroot, and hazelnut serving of mixed greens

- Cook-time TIME10 minutes
- TOTAL TIME10 minutes

INGREDIENTS

For the serving of mixed greens:

- 1 cup Puy lentils, flushed
- 2 3/4 cup sifted water
- Ocean salt
- Three cooked beetroots, cut into little shapes
- Two spring onions, finely cut
- Two tablespoons hazelnuts, generally slashed
- A bunch of crisp mints, typically cleaved
- A bunch of fresh parsley, usually cleaved

For the ginger dressing:

- The 3/4-inch shape of fresh ginger, stripped and usually cleaved
- Six tablespoons olive oil
- One teaspoon Dijon mustard
- One tablespoon apple juice vinegar
- Spot of ocean salt and crisply ground dark pepper

Directions

1. For the lentils, put them in a pan, spread with water, heat to the point of boiling the diminish the warmth and stew for around 15–20 minutes, or until all the fluid has dissipated and the lentils are not soft and still with a nibble.

2. When the lentils are cooked, exchange them to an enormous bowl and leave to cool.

3. When the lentils are cold, include the beetroot, spring onions, hazelnuts and herbs and mix until everything is consolidated.

4. For the dressing, put the ginger, mustard, oil and vinegar in a bowl and, utilizing a hand-held blender, mix until joined.

5. Sprinkle the dressing over the plate of mixed greens and serve.

10.Cauliflower steak with beans and tomatoes

- Cook TIME30 minutes
- TOTAL TIME45 minutes

INGREDIENTS

- One enormous head of cauliflower (around 2 pounds)
- 1/2 cup olive oil, isolated
- Two teaspoons fit salt, separated
- One teaspoon naturally ground dark pepper, separated
- 8 ounces green beans, cut
- Three garlic cloves, finely slashed
- 3/4 teaspoon finely ground lemon pizzazz
- 1/3 cup slashed parsley, in addition to additional for serving
- 1/3 cup panko (Japanese breadcrumbs)
- 1/4 cup naturally grated Parmesan
- 1 (15-ounce) can white beans, flushed, depleted
- 1 cup brilliant or red cherry tomatoes (around 6 ounces), divided
- Three tablespoons mayonnaise
- One teaspoon Dijon mustard

Directions

Mastermind racks in the centre and upper third of broiler; preheat to 425°F. Expel leaves and trim stem end of cauliflower, leaving centre flawless. Spot cauliflower centre side down on a work surface. Utilizing a vast blade, cut in the middle start to finish to yield 2 (1") "steaks"; save remaining cauliflower for another utilization. Spot cauliflower on a rimmed preparing sheet. Brush the two sides with 1 Tbsp. Oil; season with 1/4 tsp. Salt and 1/4 tsp. Pepper. Broil on the centre rack, turning partially through, until cauliflower is delicate and sautéed, around 30 minutes.
In the meantime, hurl green beans with 1 Tbsp. Oil, 1/2 tsp. Salt, and 1/4 tsp. Pepper on another rimmed preparing sheet. Orchestrate in a single layer, at that point cook in the upper third of broiler until green beans start to decay, around 15 minutes.
Whisk garlic, lemon pizzazz, 1/3 cup parsley, and staying 6 Tbsp. Oil, 1/4 tsp. Salt, and 1/2 tsp. Pepper in a medium bowl until smooth. Move half of the blend to another medium bowl. Add panko and Parmesan to initially bowl and blend in with your hands. Add white beans and tomatoes to second bowl and hurl to cover. Whisk mayonnaise and mustard in a little bowl.
Expel sheets from broiler. Spread mayonnaise blend over cauliflower. Sprinkle 1/4 cup panko blend equally over cauliflower. Add white bean blend to a sheet with green beans and hurl to consolidate. Return sheets to grill and keep on cooking until white beans start to fresh and panko beating begins to darker, 5–7 minutes more. Gap cauliflower, green beans, white beans, and tomatoes among plates. Top with parsley.

Cooks' Note

To cut huge, 1" "steaks" from a head of cauliflower, the inside root must stay flawless. To serve 4, utilize two enormous heads of cauliflower. Broil remaining cauliflower nearby "steaks" or fuse in soup, serving of mixed greens, or another utilization. For a vegetarian variant, swap in veggie lover mayonnaise for standard mayonnaise.

11.Lettuce wraps with smoked trout

- cook time: 15min

INGREDIENTS

- Two medium carrots, stripped
- 1/2 unpeeled English nursery cucumber (don't evacuate seeds)
- 1/4 cup daintily cut shallots
- 1/4 cup daintily cut jalapeño chiles with seeds (ideally red; around two huge)
- Two tablespoons new lime juice or unseasoned rice vinegar
- One tablespoon sugar
- One tablespoon fish sauce
- Two 4.5-ounce bundles skinless smoked trout fillets, ** broken into scaled-down pieces (around 2 cups)
- 1 cup diced grape tomatoes
- 1/2 cup entire new mint leaves
- 1/2 cup little full fresh basil leaves
- 16 low to medium internal leaves of romaine lettuce (from around two hearts of romaine)
- 1/3 cup (about) Asian sweet bean stew sauce***
- 1/4 cup finely cleaved daintily salted dry-broiled peanuts

Directions

Utilizing vegetable peeler, shave carrots and cucumber the long way into strips. Cut strips into 3-inch-long areas, at that point cut segments into matchstick-size pieces. A spot in a massive bowl. Include shallots, jalapeños, lime squeeze, sugar, and fish sauce; let marinate 30 minutes at room temperature.

Add trout pieces and tomatoes to vegetable blend and hurl to mix. Move trout-vegetable combination to a large strainer and channel off fluid. Return trout-vegetable mixture to the same bowl; include mint and basil and hurl to mix. Mastermind lettuce leaves one huge platter. Partition trout-vegetable serving of mixed greens among lettuce leaves shower sweet stew sauce over every plate of mixed greens and sprinkle with peanuts.

12.Salmon with zucchini pasta and pesto

Cook-time 20 minutes

INGREDIENTS

- 2 solidified salmon steaks (fly into the sink early to defrost, include warm water if vacuum fixed) or crisp if you can get it
- One medium to huge zucchini
- One avocado
- 1/4 cup ground parmesan
- One tablespoon of pesto (I purchase a without gluten one)
- a large portion of a lemon
- One tablespoon of dark pepper (decrease if not such a devotee of pepper)
- a spiraliser, mandolin or sharp blade
- One lemon

Directions

In the first place, pop the salmon in the grill at 180 degrees Celsius for 20 minutes, I season with some lemon squeeze and pepper, don't hesitate to include claim flavouring - Italian flavours function admirably right now, (tomato, pepper, garlic).

Make fine noodles out of your zucchini utilizing the spiraliser, mandolin or using an exceptionally sharp blade cut it lengthways, and afterwards lengthways once more. At that point make flimsy linguine formed cuts if utilizing a blade.

Crush the avocado with the lemon juice, dark pepper, and pesto and put in a safe spot.

When the salmon is cooked through (effectively drops) pop your zoodles on singular plates and top with the avocado blend and salmon. Finish everything off with parmesan and additional pesto on the off chance that you need. Appreciate :)

Choices: take out the avocado, and hamburger it up with destroyed red cabbage, cut cherry tomatoes, keep the pesto and lemon as dressing or change things up for olive oil and balsamic. Yum.

On the off chance that you are setting off to a BBQ, this could be a decent summer warm plate of mixed greens alternative, separate the salmon into pieces, cut the zoodles into shorter lengths, hurl everything together and serve.

13. Simmered cauliflower, fennel, and ginger soup

- cook time: 20min

INGREDIENTS

- 1 red onion quartered
- Four garlic cloves
- ½ head enormous cauliflower (cut into florets)
- Two fennel bulbs slashed and cored
- 500 gems load of decision
- Three tbs hummus (discretionary, I had this in the ice chest)
- 1 TBS Golden Gut Blend (or utilize 1 tsp turmeric and squeeze cinnamon and dark pepper)
- 1 tsp sage leaves
- squeeze fennel seeds
- Two tbs wheat-free tamari
- Two tbs lemon
- One handle ginger (stripped)

Directions

Preheat grill to 200 degrees Celsius

On a heating plate place red onion, garlic cloves, cauliflower and the fennel.

Heat for 30-35 minutes until firm.

Expel from the grill and spot in a blender with residual INGREDIENTS.

Mix until rich.

Fill substantial bottomed pot and spot on stovetop.

Warmth through on low to permit flavours to merge.

Season to taste.

Let cool marginally and serve warm.

Design with fennel fronds.

Glad cooking,

14. Lentil and chicken soup with sweet potato

- Cook TIME25 minutes
- TOTAL TIME35 minutes

INGREDIENTS

- One cooked chicken corpse (from 1 locally acquired rotisserie chicken or natively constructed broil chicken)
- 1 lb. sweet potatoes (around two medium), stripped, cut into 1" pieces
- 3/4 cup French lentils (about five oz.), washed
- 1 tsp. genuine salt, in addition to additional
- 2 Tbsp. extra-virgin olive oil
- Ten celery stalks, cut on the predisposition into 1/4" cuts
- Six garlic cloves, daintily cut
- 1/2 cups destroyed cooked chicken (from 1/2 of a locally acquired rotisserie chicken or custom made meal chicken)
- 1/2 head escarole, cut into reduced down pieces
- 1/2 cup finely slashed dill
- 2 Tbsp. crisp lemon juice

Directions

Spot chicken cadaver, potatoes, lentils, and 1 tsp. Salt in a huge pot. Spread with 8 cups water. Heat to the point of boiling over high warmth, skimming off any foam, at that point decrease warmth to medium-low and stew until potatoes are fork delicate and lentils are cooked through, 10–12 minutes. Dispose of a chicken cadaver.

In the interim, heat oil in a large substantial skillet over medium-high. Include celery and garlic and cook, regularly blending, until celery and garlic are daintily brilliant dark-coloured and delicate, around 12 minutes.

Mix celery, garlic, destroyed chicken, and escarole into soup and cook, mixing sporadically, until escarole is withered, around 5 minutes. Expel from heat. Mix in dill and lemon juice; season soup with salt.

15.Salmon with greens and cauliflower rice

- cook time: 15min

INGREDIENTS

- Two salmon filets, economically sourced or natural
- 10 to 12 Brussels grows, hacked into equal parts
- One pack kale washed and destroyed
- ½ head cauliflower, beat into cauliflower rice (you can utilize an entire cauliflower head if you wish)
- Three tablespoons olive or coconut oil
- One teaspoon curry powder
- Himalayan salt
- For marinade
- ¼ cup tamari sauce
- One teaspoon Dijon mustard
- One teaspoon sesame oil
- One teaspoon nectar or maple syrup (discretionary)
- One tablespoon sesame seeds

Directions

Preheat stove to 350°F.

Line a preparing plate and include cleaved Brussels grows. Coat with one tablespoon oil and season with salt. Add to barbecue and dish for 20 minutes.

In the interim, make the marinade by joining all INGREDIENTS in a bowl and racing until consolidated.

Evacuate Brussels grows following 20 minutes and add salmon filets to the heating plate. Spoon marinade over salmon filets and come back to stove for a further 13 to 15 minutes, or until salmon is cooked just as you would prefer.

While salmon is cooking, heat a skillet over medium-high warmth and include one tablespoon oil. Include kale and sauté until withered (2 to 3 minutes). Expel from the dish and put in a safe spot.

Warmth remaining oil in a dish and include cauliflower rice. Season with one teaspoon curry powder and salt and sauté until cooked (2 to 3 minutes).

Expel salmon and Brussels grows from stove and separation into two dishes. Include sautéed kale and cauliflower rice to bowls.

16.Shrimp and vegetable curry

- Planning Time 10 minutes
- Cook Time 15 minutes

INGREDIENTS

- 3 TBSP margarine or coconut oil
- One onion cut
- 1 cup of coconut milk
- 1-3 tsp curry powder
- 1 lb shrimp tails evacuated
- One pack solidified cauliflower or other solidified veggies of decision

Guidelines

Liquefy spread or oil in a skillet and include cut onion.

Saute onion until it is marginally delicate.

In the meantime, steam vegetables.

At the point when the onion is mellowed include coconut milk, curry flavouring, and different flavours whenever wanted.

Cook a few minutes to consolidate flavours.

Include defrosted shrimp and cook roughly 5 minutes or until shrimp are cooked

Present with steamed veggies of decision bested with spread and plate of mixed greens with handcrafted dressing.

Notes

I have a few flavouring mixes plans accessible, just as one for handcrafted curry powder.

17.Vegan stew

- Planning Time: 20 mins
- Cook Time: 40 mins

INGREDIENTS

- Two tablespoons extra-virgin olive oil
- One medium red onion, hacked
- One huge red ringer pepper slashed
- Two medium carrots, hacked
- Two ribs celery, hacked
- ½ teaspoon salt, separated
- Four cloves garlic, squeezed or minced
- Two tablespoons stew powder*
- Two teaspoons ground cumin
- 1 ½ teaspoon smoked paprika*
- One teaspoon dried oregano
- One huge can (28 ounces) or two little jars (15 ounces each) diced tomatoes**, with their juices
- Two jars (15 ounces each) dark beans, washed and depleted
- One can (15 ounces) pinto beans, rinsed and depleted
- 2 cups vegetable soup or water
- One inlet leaf
- Two tablespoons hacked new cilantro, in addition to additional for embellishing
- 1 to 2 teaspoons sherry vinegar or red wine vinegar or lime juice, to taste

Directions

In a large Dutch broiler or overwhelming bottomed pot over medium warmth, warm the olive oil until shining. Include the hacked onion, chime pepper, carrot, celery and ¼ teaspoon of the salt. Mix to consolidate and cook, mixing every so often, until the vegetables are delicate and the onion is translucent around 7 to 10 minutes.

Include the garlic, bean stew powder, cumin, smoked paprika and oregano. Cook until fragrant while blending continually, around one moment.

Include the diced tomatoes and their juices, the depleted dark beans and pinto beans, vegetable stock and narrows leaf. Mix to consolidate and let the blend go to a stew. Keep cooking, blending every so often and decreasing warmth as essential to keep up a delicate stew, for 30 minutes. Expel the casserole from the heat.

For the best surface and flavour, move 1 ½ cups of the stew to a blender, making a point to get a portion of the fluid bit. Safely affix the cover and mix until smooth (keep an eye out for hot steam), at that point empty the mixed blend once again into the pot. (Or then again, you can combine the bean stew quickly with a drenching blender, or squash the casserole with a potato masher until it arrives at a thicker, more stew-like consistency.)

Include the cleaved cilantro, mix to mix, and afterwards blend in the vinegar, to taste. Add salt to taste, as well I included ¼ teaspoon more now. Gap the blend into unique dishes and present with trimmings of your decision. This bean stew will keep well in the cooler for around four days, or you can freeze it for longer-term stockpiling.

NOTES

Plans counselled during the creation of this formula: vegan bean stew with winter vegetables (The New York Times), veggie lover bean stew (Saveur) and winter vegetable stew (Food and Wine).

18.Salmon cakes

- Prep: 30 min

INGREDIENTS

- 1/2-pound new salmon
- Great olive oil
- Legitimate salt and naturally ground dark pepper
- Four tablespoons unsalted spread
- 3/4 cup little diced red onion (1 little onion)
- 1/2 cups little diced celery (4 stalks)
- 1/2 cup little diced red ringer pepper (1 little pepper)
- 1/2 cup little diced yellow ringer pepper (1 little pepper)
- 1/4 cup minced crisp level leaf parsley
- One tablespoon escapades, depleted
- 1/4 teaspoon hot sauce (prescribed: Tabasco)
- 1/2 teaspoon Worcestershire sauce
- 1/2 teaspoons crab bubble flavouring (prescribed: Old Bay)
- 3 cups stale bread, outside layers, expelled
- 1/2 cup great mayonnaise
- Two teaspoons Dijon mustard
- Two extra-enormous eggs, daintily beaten

Directions

Preheat the grill to 350 degrees F.

Spot the salmon on a sheet skillet, skin side down. Brush with olive oil and sprinkle with salt and pepper. Broil for 15 to 20 minutes, until simply cooked. Expel from the broiler and spread firmly with aluminium foil. Permit to rest for 10 minutes and refrigerate until cold.

Then, place two tablespoons of the spread, two tablespoons olive oil, the onion, celery, red and yellow ringer peppers, parsley, tricks, hot sauce, Worcestershire sauce, crab bubble flavouring, 1/2 teaspoon salt, and 1/2 teaspoon pepper in an enormous saute skillet over medium-low warmth and cook until the vegetables are delicate, roughly 15 to 20 minutes. Cool to room temperature.

Fellowship cuts in pieces and procedure the bread in a nourishment processor fitted with a steel edge. You ought to have around 1 cup of bread pieces. Spot the bread morsels on a sheet dish and toast in the stove for 5 minutes until daintily carmelized, hurling every so often.

Piece the chilled salmon into a large bowl. Include the bread scraps, mayonnaise, mustard, and eggs. Include the vegetable blend and blend well. Spread and chill in the cooler for 30 minutes. Shape into 10 (2 1/2 to 3-ounce) cakes.

Warmth the staying two tablespoons spread and two tablespoons olive oil in a large saute container over medium heat. In bunches, include the salmon cakes and fry for 3 to 4 minutes on each side, until caramelized. Channel on paper towels; keep them warm in a preheated 250-degree F grill and serve hot.

19. Force balls

- cook time: 30min

INGRIDENTS

- 1/2 cup (10g) PUFFED MILLET
- 1 cup (20g) PUFFED KAMUT or PUFFED RICE
- 1/2 cup (90g) diced DRIED PLUMS (prunes; see Note)
- 1/3 cup (60g) SEMISWEET CHOCOLATE CHIPS
- 1/4 cup (35g) SESAME SEEDS
- 1/3 cup (80g) SUNFLOWER BUTTER, at room temperature
- 1/2 cup (125ml) HONEY
- 3/4 cup (40g) destroyed unsweetened COCONUT

Directions

1. In a considerable bowl, hurl together the puffed millet and puffed Kamut or rice. Include the dried plums, chocolate chips, and sesame seeds.

2. Mix in the sunflower spread and the nectar. You ought to have a decent clingy mess! Spread the bowl with cling wrap and refrigerate for 30 minutes.

3. Spot the coconut in a little bowl. Utilizing a tablespoon, scoop the blend and structure it into 1-inch (2.5cm) balls with your hands. Roll the balls in the coconut and move to a holder. You can store the force balls in the cooler for as long as a multi-week, or in the cooler in a zip-top cooler sack for as long as a multi-month, yet I wager they won't keep going that long!

Note:

There's an item from Sunsweet called Plum Amazing that is just diced dried plums. Since they can be annoyingly clingy to cleave up, I discover the predicted ones accommodating for assembling this formula rapidly.

20.Chia seed pudding

- Cook time 10mins

INGREDIENTS

- One 13.5-ounce can light coconut milk
- Three tablespoons chia seeds
- Three tablespoons unadulterated maple syrup
- 1/2 cup crisp pineapple lumps
- Two medium kiwis, stripped and cut
- 1/4 cup raspberries
- Two tablespoons simmered almonds, slashed

Directions

Unique hardware: four 8-ounce glass containers with covers.

Mix the coconut milk, chia seeds and maple syrup in a medium bowl. Separation the blend equitably among four 8-ounce glass containers. Screw on the tops, and refrigerate medium-term, secured, to permit the seeds to be full and the mixture to thicken into a free pudding.

Organize the pineapples, kiwis, raspberries and almonds in discrete layers over the pudding. Spread with the top, and keep refrigerated for as long as one day.

21.Turmeric nachos

- cook time: 10mins

INGREDIENTS

- Two tomatoes, diced
- One cucumber, diced
- Nachos chips
- 100 g (31/2 oz/1 cup) almond dinner
- One huge natural egg
- One teaspoon turmeric
- 1/4 teaspoon cumin
- 1/4 teaspoon coriander
- One teaspoon ground orange get-up-and-go
- One teaspoon Celtic ocean salt

Directions

To cause the chips, to preheat the stove to 180°C (350°F/Gas 4).

Spot all the chip INGREDIENTS in a considerable bowl and blend in with a wooden spoon to shape a mixture.

Spot the batter on a perfect work surface between two bits of heating paper. Turn the dough out until it is 2 mm (1/16 inch) thick.

Evacuate the top bit of preparing paper and move the mixture and base bit of heating paper to a heating plate. Utilizing a sharp blade, profoundly score the batter each 3 cm (11/4 inch), at that point do the other way likewise, so you structure squares.

Heat in the grill for 12 minutes.

Permit to cool before breaking them separated.

To amass the nachos, place the Nachos chips on a slashing board, and top with the rest of the INGREDIENTS.

Any extra chips will keep in a water/air proof compartment for as long as three days.

22.Matcha smoothie bowl

- Planning TIME: 5 minutes
- Complete TIME: 5 minutes

INGREDIENTS

- SMOOTHIE
- Two stripped, cut and solidified ready bananas (~120 g each)
- 1/4 cup hacked available pineapple (discretionary/solidified is ideal)
- 3/4 - 1 cup light coconut milk (canned or carton)
- 2 tsp matcha green tea powder (see our Matcha Review!)
- One piling cup natural spinach or kale (I like to hold up mine to make the smoothie colder!)

INGREDIENTS discretionary

- New berries
- Coconut chip
- Banana cuts
- Chia Seeds
- Fragmented broiled almonds

Directions

Include solidified banana cuts, pineapple (discretionary), the lesser measure of coconut milk (3/4 cup or 180 ml as the unique formula is composed/change if adjusting cluster size), matcha powder, and spinach to a blender and mix on high until velvety and smooth.

Include just like a lot of coconut milk as you have to enable it to mix. As I would see it, you need this smoothie somewhere close to scoopable and drinkable.

Taste and alter season varying, including more banana (or a pinch of maple syrup or stevia) for sweetness, matcha for progressively exceptional green tea flavour, or coconut milk for richness (however including more matcha powder includes more caffeine, so utilize your best carefulness). Pineapple will consist of somewhat tart/tang, so add more whenever wanted.

The gap between two serving bowls (sum as the unique formula is composed/change if adjusting group size) and top with wanted garnishes (discretionary). I went with new raspberries, chia seeds, and coconut piece. Bananas would make a rich embellishment also. Best when crisp, however, remains to keep all-around fixed in the cooler as long as 24 hours.

Recipes For Lunch

23.Devilled egg salad

INGREDIENTS:

- 12 enormous eggs
- 1/4 cup slashed green onion
- 1/2 cup slashed celery
- 1/2 cup slashed red chime pepper
- 2 tablespoons Dijon mustard
- 1/3 cup mayonnaise
- 1 tablespoon juice, white wine or sherry vinegar
- 1/4 teaspoon Tabasco or other hot sauce (pretty much to taste)
- 1/2 teaspoon paprika (pretty much to taste)
- 1/2 teaspoon dark pepper (pretty much to taste)
- 1/4 teaspoon salt (more to taste)

INSTRUCTIONS:

Hard heat up the eggs: The simplest method to make hard bubbled eggs that are anything but difficult to strip is to steam them. Fill a pan with 1 inch of water and addition a steamer bushel. (On the off chance that you don't have a steamer bushel, that is alright.)

Heat the water to the point of boiling, delicately place the eggs in the steamer bin or straightforwardly in the pan. Spread the pot. Set your clock for 15 minutes. Evacuate eggs and set in frigid virus water to cool.

Prep the eggs and veggies: Chop the eggs coarsely and put them into a huge bowl. Include the green onion, celery, and red chime pepper.

Make the plate of mixed greens: In little bowl, combine the mayo, mustard, vinegar, and Tabasco. Tenderly mix the mayo dressing into the bowl with the eggs and vegetables. Include the paprika and salt and dark pepper. Change seasonings to taste.

24.Pounded chickpea salad
INGREDIENTS:

- 1 avocado
- 1/2 crisp lemon
- 1 can chickpeas depleted (19 oz)
- 1/4 cup cut red onion
- 2 cups grape tomatoes cut
- 2 cups diced cucumber
- 1/2 cup crisp parsley
- 3/4 cup diced green chime pepper

Dressing

- 1/4 cup olive oil
- 2 tablespoons red wine vinegar
- 1/2 teaspoon cumin
- salt and pepper

INSTRUCTIONS:

Cut avocado into 3D squares and spot in bowl. Press the juice from 1/2 lemon over the avocado and delicately mix to consolidate.

Include remaining serving of mixed greens ingredients and delicately hurl to join. Refrigerate at any rate one hour before serving.

25.Strawberry and goat cheese salad

INGREDIENTS:

- 1-pound crisp strawberries, diced
- Discretionary: 1 to 2 teaspoons nectar or maple syrup, to taste
- 2 ounces disintegrated goat cheddar (about ½ cup)
- ¼ cup cleaved crisp basil, in addition to a couple of little basil leaves for embellish
- 1 tablespoon extra-virgin olive oil
- 1 tablespoon thick balsamic vinegar*
- ½ teaspoon Maldon flaky ocean salt or an inadequate ¼ teaspoon fine ocean salt
- Crisply ground dark pepper

INSTRUCTIONS:

Spread the diced strawberries over a medium serving platter or shallow serving bowl. In the event that the strawberries aren't sufficiently sweet exactly as you would prefer, hurl them with a touch of nectar or maple syrup.

Sprinkle the disintegrated goat cheddar over the strawberries, trailed by the hacked basil. Shower the olive oil and balsamic vinegar on top.

Polish off the plate of mixed greens with the salt, a couple of bits of crisply ground dark pepper, and the saved basil leaves. For the most excellent introduction, serve the plate of mixed greens speedily. Scraps will keep well in the fridge, however, for around 3 days.

26.Dark bean freezer burritos

INGREDIENTS:

- 2 Tbsp additional virgin olive oil
- 1 enormous yellow onion diced
- 4 cloves garlic squashed or minced
- 1 jalapeño seeded and finely minced
- 1 enormous red chime pepper diced
- 1 medium zucchini diced
- 1 cup corn parts new, solidified, or canned are for the most part fine
- 1 tomato dice
- 1 cup cooked quinoa from around 1/2 cup uncooked
- 3 cups dark beans approx. two 14oz jars
- 1 Tbsp ground cumin
- 1 tsp hot smoked paprika
- 1 tsp bean stew powder
- 1 tsp salt
- 1/2 bundle cilantro cleaved
- 1 cup destroyed cheddar discretionary
- 6 enormous entire wheat tortillas

INSTRUCTIONS:

Start by getting the entirety of your slashing off the beaten path, it'll assist everything with meeting up quicker once you begin cooking. Hack the onion, pound the garlic, mince the jalapeño, dice the zucchini and red pepper, and set everything into little dishes or on plates. Presently you're all set!

Warmth the oil in an enormous skillet over medium-high warmth.

Include the onions and sauté for around 5 minutes, blending much of the time, until the onions are delicate and starting to take on a touch of shading.

Include the garlic and jalapeños and sauté for around 2 minutes more.

Presently include the zucchini and red pepper and sauté for 8-10 minutes. The vegetables ought to be relaxed yet not soft, and simply beginning to dark colored.

Now include the corn, and tomato and sauté for 2-3 minutes, until the blend is very much warmed.

Include the quinoa, dark beans, cumin, smoked paprika, stew, and salt. Mix to join well.

Taste, and modify seasonings if vital. Mix in the cilantro, and expel from the warmth.

Presently you're good to go! Gap the burrito filling between the six tortillas (or more in the event that you need littler burritos), sprinkle with cheddar whenever wanted, and roll!

To freeze the burritos, wrap separately in foil or material paper, and spot in a solitary layer in the cooler.

To make the most of your cooler burrito you can prepare and haul one out of the cooler the prior night, or simply snatch one directly from the cooler toward the beginning of the day. I let mine defrost close to me around my work area, at that point heat it up in the workplace microwave at noon. Appreciate

27.Creamy garbano salad

INGREDIENTS:

- Plate of mixed greens
- 2 14 oz jars Chickpeas
- 3/4 cup Carrot little shakers
- 3/4 cup Celery little shakers
- 3/4 cup Bell Pepper Small shakers
- 1 Scallion hacked
- 1/4 cup Red Onion little shakers
- 1/2 Large Avocado
- 6 oz smooth tofu
- 1 Tbsp Apple Cider Vinegar
- 1 Tbsp Lemon Juice
- 1 Tbsp Dijon Mustard
- 1 Tbsp Sweet Relish
- 1/4 tsp Smoked Paprika
- 1/4 tsp Celery seeds
- 1/4 tsp Black Pepper
- 1/4 tsp Mustard powder
- Ocean salt to taste
- Sandwich Fix'ns
- Grown Whole Grain Bread
- Cut Roma Tomatoes
- Spread Lettuce

INSTRUCTIONS:

Get ready and slash your carrots, celery, chime pepper, red onion and scallion and spot in a little blending bowl. Put In a safe spot.

Utilizing a little submersion blender or nourishment processor, mix the avocado, tofu, apple juice vinegar, lemon juice, and mustard until smooth.

Strain and wash your garbanzos, and spot in a medium blending bowl. With a potato masher or a fork squash the beans until most are separated and it begins to take after fish plate of mixed greens. You don't need it to be smooth however finished and stout. Season the beans with a spot of salt and pepper.

Include the cleaved vegetables, avocado-tofu cream, and the rest of the flavors and relish and blend well. Taste and alter as indicated by your inclination.

28.Slight bistro box

The incredible thing about these bistro boxes is that you can include whatever you might want!

Bistro Snack Box 1: Cucumber cuts, 1 carrot (stripped and cut), 1 cut celery stalk, side of hummus.

1 hard bubbled egg, 1 ounce of cubed cheddar, 1 cup grapes, 4 Tricots (or wafers of decision).

Cold Protein Packed Bistro Box - figure out how to make your own bite boxes - effectively and rapidly! These two-choice bistros enclose meets up minutes and are flawless as a post-exercise nibble, for feast prepared snacks, or on the off chance that you live in a hurry!

Bistro Snack Box 2: 1 mandarin orange, 1 cup of berries, 1 hard bubbled egg, 1/4 cup of almonds, 1/2 cup curds.

Cold Protein Packed Bistro Box - figure out how to make your own bite boxes - effectively and rapidly! These two choice bistro confines meet up minutes and are impeccable as a post-exercise nibble, for supper prepared snacks, or in the event that you live in a hurry!

The alternatives are perpetual!

Not an aficionado of the natural product imagined or recorded? Include your preferred product! Raspberries, peaches, apple cuts, banana cuts, pineapple pieces, and so on.

Swap the curds for greek or skyr yogurt.

Not an aficionado of almonds? Swap for pecans, walnuts, pistachios, cashews. Simply ensure they are crude or possibly gently salted.

29. Carrot noodles with ginger lime peanut sauce

INGREDIENTS:

For the carrot pasta:

- 5 huge carrots, stripped and julienned or spiraled into slim strips
- 1/3 cup (50g) cooked cashews
- 2 tablespoons new cilantro, finely hacked

For the ginger-peanut sauce:

- 2 tablespoons rich nutty spread
- 4 tablespoons ordinary coconut milk
- Squeeze cayenne pepper
- 2 huge cloves garlic, finely hacked
- 1 tablespoon new ginger, stripped and ground
- 1 tablespoon lime juice
- Salt, to taste

INSTRUCTIONS:

Consolidate all sauce ingredients in a little bowl and combine until smooth and rich and put in a safe spot while you julienne/spiralize the carrots.

In a huge serving bowl, tenderly hurl the carrots and sauce together until equally covered. Top with broiled cashews (or peanuts) and newly hacked cilantro.

30.Tequila flank steak fajita salad

INGREDIENTS:

- TEQUILA LIME FLANK STEAK
- 1 (2 pound, 1-inch) thick flank steak
- 1/3 cup tequila
- 1/4 cup olive oil
- 1/4 cup lime juice
- 1/2 teaspoon salt
- 1/2 teaspoon pepper
- pizzazz of 2 limes
- 1/2 red pepper, meagerly cut
- 1/2 green pepper, meagerly cut
- 1 tablespoon olive oil
- 1 head of red romaine lettuce, washed, dried and torn
- 1/2 cup dark beans
- 1/2 cup copycat chipotle corn salsa
- 1-ounce Colby jack cheddar, naturally ground
- 1 avocado, cut
- blue tortilla chips for garnish
- CHILE LIME VINAIGRETTE
- 2 tablespoons olive oil
- 1 tablespoons rice vinegar
- 1/2 tablespoon red pepper or chile oil
- 2 teaspoons nectar
- the juice of 2 limes
- a touch of salt + pepper

INSTRUCTIONS:

Whisk tequila, olive oil, lime juice, salt, pepper and lime get-up-and-go in a bowl until join. Add flank steak to a Ziplock pack or preparing dish and pour marinade ingredients over top. Marinate (in the ice chest!) for 2-24 hours, flipping steak a couple of times. At the point when you're prepared to make the plates of mixed greens, heat the grill in your broiler on the most noteworthy setting and spot a stove rack straightforwardly underneath. Sear steak for 5 minutes, flip and cook for 5 minutes more. In the event that your steak is 1/2 inches thick, this will bring about steak that is done medium-well. Let it rest for 5-10 minutes, at that point cut slight strips on an edge. You can cook the steak anyway you'd like! You can flame broil the steak whenever wanted.

While the steak is cooking/resting, heat a skillet over medium warmth and include olive oil. Include peppers with a touch of salt and pepper, hurling to cover and cook for 5-6 minutes, until marginally delicate.

To gather the serving of mixed greens, place lettuce in the bowl with a spot of salt and pepper, hurl, and spread with flank steak, dark beans, corn salsa, peppers, cheddar, avocado and tortilla chips. Top with dressing and hurl!

31.BLT pasta salad

INGREDIENTS:

- 10 cuts bacon cooked and diced; oil saved
- 12 oz pasta cooked and cooled
- 1/2 cup mayonnaise
- 3/4 cup farm dressing hand crafted farm is ideal
- 1/2 cup diced tomatoes
- 1/2 avocado diced
- 1 cup cheddar destroyed
- 1/3 cup red onion diced
- 1 cup romaine lettuce
- new parsley for decorate discretionary

INSTRUCTIONS:

Whisk together mayonnaise, farm dressing and 1 tablespoon bacon oil (discretionary).

In a huge bowl collect the pasta, tomatoes, avocado, cheddar, red onion, lettuce and bacon.

Pour the dressing over and hurl to consolidate.

Enhancement with parsley and serve.

32.Greek yogurt chicken salad

INGREDIENTS:

- Chopped chicken
- Green apple
- Red onion
- Celery
- Dried cranberries

SERVING SUGGESTIONS

Greek yogurt chicken serving of mixed greens is such an extraordinary supper prep lunch thought. You can place it in an artisan jostle and eat only that or you can pack it in a super prep compartment with more veggies, chips, and so forth. Here are some serving recommendations.

On a bit of toast

In a tortilla with lettuce

With chips or saltines

In a bit of ice burg lettuce (low carb choice!)

33.Meatballs alla parmigiana

INGREDIENTS:

For the meatballs

- 1.5lbs ground hamburger (80/20)
- 2 Tbl crisp parsley, cleaved
- 3/4 cup ground parmesan cheddar
- 1/2 cup almond flour
- 2 eggs
- 1 tsp fit salt
- 1/4 tsp ground dark pepper
- 1/4 tsp garlic powder
- 1 tsp dried onion drops
- 1/4 tsp dried oregano
- 1/2 cup warm water
- For the Parmigiana
- 1 cup simple keto marinara sauce (or any sugar free locally acquired marinara)
- 4 oz mozzarella cheddar

Guidelines:

Join the entirety of the meatball fixings in a huge bowl and blend well.

Structure into fifteen 2″ meatballs.

Prepare at 350 degrees (F) for 20 minutes OR fry in an enormous skillet over medium warmth until cooked through. Ace tip – have a go at searing in bacon oil in the event that you have any – it includes another degree of flavor. Fricasseeing produces the brilliant dark colored shading appeared in the photographs above.

For the Parmigiana:

Spot the cooked meatballs in a stove safe dish.

Spoon roughly 1 Tbl sauce over every meatball.

Spread with roughly 1/4 oz of mozzarella cheddar each.

Prepare at 350 degrees (F) for 20 minutes (40 minutes if meatballs are solidified) or until warmed through and the cheddar is brilliant.

Embellishment with new parsley whenever wanted.

34. Quinoa and sweet potato cakes

INGREDIENTS:

- 3/4 cup quinoa, flushed
- 2 Tbsp olive oil, in addition to additional for fricasseeing
- 1 little onion, diced
- 2 garlic cloves, minced
- 2 cups ground sweet potato
- 1 tsp salt
- 1/4 tsp allspice
- 1/2 tsp smoked paprika
- 1/2 tsp oregano
- 2 eggs
- 1/2 cup breadcrumbs
- 1/2 cup ground parmesan cheddar
- 2 Tbsp finely cleaved cilantro
- Green onions and cabbage, as topping

Guidelines:

Cook the quinoa as indicated by headings, and put aside to cool.

As the quinoa is cooking, heat 2 Tbsp olive oil in an enormous skillet.

In the skillet, cook the onion and garlic for a couple of moments, until starting to mellow.

Include the ground sweet potato and the entirety of the flavors. Cook for an additional 3 minutes.

Expel from warmth, and permit to sufficiently cool to deal with before proceeding.

In an enormous bowl, whisk together the eggs, breadcrumbs, cheddar, and cilantro, at that point include the cooled quinoa and vegetable blend. Blend to completely join.

In a substantial skillet over medium warmth, heat increasingly olive oil before including the hitter in little touches (or formed into little patties). Cook until brilliant on each side, around 2 minutes.

Serve on a bed of greens or cabbage, embellished with green onions.

35.Cold soba with miso dressing

INGREDIENTS:

- 6oz buckwheat Soba noodles
- 1/2 cups destroyed carrots
- 1 cup solidified shelled edamame, defrosted
- 2 Persian cucumbers, cut
- 1 cup hacked cilantro
- 1/4 cup sesame seeds
- 2 tbsp dark sesame seeds
- White Miso Dressing (makes 2 cups)
- 2/3 cup white miso glue
- Juice of 2 medium size lemons
- 4 tbsp rice vinegar
- 4 tbsp additional virgin olive oil
- 4 tbsp squeezed orange
- 2 tbsp new ground ginger
- 2 tbsp maple syrup

Directions:

Cook soba noodles as per the guidelines in the bundling (make a point not to overcook them or they will get sticky and remain together). Channel well and move to an enormous bowl

Include destroyed carrots, edamame, cucumber, cilantro and sesame seeds

To set up the dressing, consolidate every one of the fixings in a blender. Mix until smooth

Pour wanted measure of dressing over the noodles (we utilized about a cup and a half)

36.BLT spring rolls

INGRIDENTS:

- new lettuce, torn pieces or slashed
- 1 medium tomato (seeded and cut 1/4" thick)
- 6 pieces bacon, cooked
- new basil, mint or different herbs
- rice paper
- avocado cuts, discretionary

SESAME-SOY DIPPING SAUCE

- 1/4 cup Soy Sauce
- 1/4 cup cold water
- 1 Tablespoon Mayonnaise (discretionary, this makes the plunge velvety)
- 1 teaspoon new Lime Juice
- 1 teaspoon Sesame Oil
- 1 teaspoon sriracha sauce or any hot sauce (discretionary)

Guidelines:

37.SPRING ROLL DIRECTIONS

In enormous bowl, fill it with water and make it warm by including heated water. Tenderly dunk each rice paper wrapper in warm water for a couple of moments until soggy. Don't over drench the rice paper, it will keep engrossing the water on its surface in the wake of expelling from the high temp water. Spot rice paper on plate or working surface. As rice paper retains the water and turn out to be all the more delicate and malleable (around 10-20 seconds, contingent upon wrappers and water temp.), start to include the fillings.

On the 1/3 segment of the rice paper wrapper nearest to you, begin layering your fillings of lettuce, tomatoes and bacon. You can simply have 1 bacon for each spring roll however in the event that you need to make it extra delightful and wanton, include 2 cuts of bacon.

Begin rolling the wrapper once again the fillings from you, tucking and rolling the wrapper with your fingers, ensuring every one of the fillings stay tight and round inside the rice paper wrapper.

Serve promptly, or spread with saran wrap to eat a couple of hours after the fact.

38. Alfredo zucchini pasta

INGRIDENTS:

- 2 medium zucchinis spiralized
- 1-2 TB Vegan Parmesan (discretionary)
- Fast Alfredo Sauce
- 1/2 cup crude cashews drenched for a couple of hours or in bubbling water for 10 minutes
- 2 TB lemon juice
- 3 TB nourishing yeast
- 2 tsp white miso (can sub tamari, soy sauce, or coconut aminos)
- 1 tsp onion powder
- 1/2 tsp garlic powder
- 1/4-1/2 cup water

Guidelines:

Spiralize zucchini noodles.

Add all alfredo fixings to a fast blender (beginning with 1/4 cup of water) and mix until smooth. In the event that your sauce is excessively thick, include more water a tablespoon at once until you get the consistency you're searching for.

Top zucchini noodles with alfredo sauce and on the off chance that you'd like, some vegetarian pram.

39.Quinoa burrito bowls

INGREDIENTS:

- 1 formula Cilantro Lime Quinoa
- For the dark beans:
- 1 can dark beans
- 1 teaspoon ground cumin
- 1 teaspoon dried oregano
- salt, to taste

For the cherry tomato pico de gallo:

- 1 dry 16 ounces cherry or grape tomatoes, quartered
- 1/2 cup diced red onion
- 1 Tablespoon minced jalapeno pepper , (ribs and seeds expelled, whenever wanted)
- 1/2 cup cleaved crisp cilantro
- 2 Tablespoons lime juice
- salt, to taste

For the fixings:

- cut cured jalapenos
- 1 avocado, diced

Directions

Set up the Cilantro Lime Quinoa and keep warm.

In a little sauce container, join the dark beans and their fluid with the cumin and oregano over medium warmth. Mix periodically until the beans are hot. Taste and include salt, whenever wanted.

Consolidate the elements for the cherry tomato pico de gallo in a bowl and hurl well.

To amass the burrito bowls, partition the Cilantro Lime Quinoa among four dishes. Include a fourth of the dark beans to each. Top with cherry tomato pico de gallo, cut pickled jalapenos, and avocado. Appreciate!

Note:

The entirety of the components of these dishes can be made early and amassed when prepared to eat. You can either warm the quinoa and beans, or appreciate them at room temperature. I like to cause the segments throughout the end of the week so I to can appreciate Quinoa Burrito Bowls for lunch during the week.

40.Fiery tuna salad

Change it up of fish (mine is strong white tuna fish pressed in water) to a bowl in the wake of depleting it very well of the water (or the oil) it was stuffed in.

Include your mayo, your mustard, your new dill (or your preferred herb—chives are incredible, as well), your red onion, the lemon pizzazz, and some salt and pepper. Cautiously overlay every one of the fixings together until well-joined; and either appreciate quickly, or keep in a shrouded compartment in the ice chest for later use on sandwiches, wafers, over greens, or even with simply a spoon!

41.Shredded chicken gyros

INGRIDENTS:

- 2 medium onions, cleaved
- 6 garlic cloves, minced
- 1 teaspoon lemon-pepper flavoring
- 1 teaspoon dried oregano
- 1/2 teaspoon ground allspice
- 1/2 cup water
- 1/2 cup lemon juice
- 1/4 cup red wine vinegar
- 2 tablespoons olive oil
- 2 pounds boneless skinless chicken bosoms
- 8 entire pita breads

Discretionary fixings: Tzatziki sauce, torn romaine and cut tomato, cucumber and onion

Directions:

In a 3-qt. slow cooker, consolidate initial 9 fixings; include chicken. Cook, secured, on low 3-4 hours or until chicken is delicate (a thermometer should peruse at any rate 165°).

Expel chicken from moderate cooker. Shred with 2 forks; come back to slow cooker. Utilizing tongs, place chicken blend on pita breads. Present with garnishes.

42.Pepperoni pizza loaf

INGREDIENTS:

- 1 portion (1 pound) solidified bread mixture, defrosted
- 2 enormous eggs, isolated
- 1 tablespoon ground Parmesan cheddar
- 1 tablespoon olive oil
- 1 teaspoon minced crisp parsley
- 1 teaspoon dried oregano
- 1/2 teaspoon garlic powder
- 1/4 teaspoon pepper
- 8 ounces cut pepperoni
- 2 cups destroyed part-skim mozzarella cheddar
- 1 can (4 ounces) mushroom stems and pieces, depleted
- 1/4 to 1/2 cup cured pepper rings
- 1 medium green pepper, diced
- 1 can (2-1/4 ounces) cut ready olives
- 1 can (15 ounces) pizza sauce

Directions:

Preheat stove to 350°. On a lubed preparing sheet, turn out batter into a 15x10-in. square shape. In a little bowl, consolidate the egg yolks, Parmesan cheddar, oil, parsley, oregano, garlic powder and pepper. Brush over the mixture.

Sprinkle with the pepperoni, mozzarella cheddar, mushrooms, pepper rings, green pepper and olives. Move up, jam move style, beginning with a long side; squeeze crease to seal and fold finishes under.

Position portion with crease side down; brush with egg whites. Try not to let rise. Prepare until brilliant dark colored and mixture is cooked through, 35-40 minutes. Warm the pizza sauce; present with cut portion.

Freeze choice: Freeze cooled unsliced pizza portion in uncompromising foil. To utilize, expel from cooler 30 minutes before warming. Expel from thwart and warm portion on a lubed preparing sheet in a preheated 325° broiler until warmed through. Fill in as coordinated.

43.Cashew chicken rotini salad

INGREDIENTS:

- 1 bundle (16 ounces) winding or rotini pasta
- 4 cups cubed cooked chicken
- 1 can (20 ounces) pineapple goodies, depleted
- 1-1/2 cups cut celery
- 3/4 cup daintily cut green onions
- 1 cup seedless red grapes
- 1 cup seedless green grapes
- 1 bundle (5 ounces) dried cranberries
- 1 cup farm plate of mixed greens dressing
- 3/4 cup mayonnaise
- 2 cups salted cashews

Directions:

Cook pasta as per bundle bearings. In the meantime, in a huge bowl, join the chicken, pineapple, celery, onions, grapes and cranberries. Channel pasta and flush in chilly water; mix into chicken blend.

In a little bowl, whisk the farm dressing and mayonnaise. Pour over plate of mixed greens and hurl to cover. Cover and refrigerate for at any rate 60 minutes. Just before serving, mix in cashews.

44.Honey lime roasted chicken

INGREDIENTS:

- 1 entire simmering chicken (5 to 6 pounds)
- 1/2 cup lime juice
- 1/4 cup nectar
- 1 tablespoon stone-ground mustard or fiery darker mustard
- 1 teaspoon salt
- 1 teaspoon ground cumin

Guidelines:

Cautiously slacken the skin from the whole chicken. Spot bosom side up on a rack in a simmering skillet. In a little bowl, whisk the lime juice, nectar, mustard, salt and cumin.

Utilizing a turkey baster, season under the chicken skin with 1/3 cup lime juice blend. Tie drumsticks together. Pour remaining lime juice blend over chicken.

Broil until a thermometer embedded in thickest piece of thigh peruses 170°-175°, 2-2-1/2 hours. (Spread freely with foil if chicken tans too immediately.) Let represent 10 minutes before cutting. Whenever wanted, expel and dispose of skin before serving.

45.Quinoa turkey chicken

INGRIDENTS:

- 1 cup quinoa, flushed
- 3-1/2 cups water, isolated
- 1/2-pound lean ground turkey
- 1 enormous sweet onion, slashed
- 1 medium sweet red pepper, slashed
- 4 garlic cloves, minced
- 1 tablespoon bean stew powder
- 1 tablespoon ground cumin
- 1/2 teaspoon ground cinnamon
- 2 jars (15 ounces each) dark beans, flushed and depleted
- 1 can (28 ounces) squashed tomatoes
- 1 medium zucchini, slashed
- 1 chipotle pepper in adobo sauce, slashed
- 1 tablespoon adobo sauce
- 1 narrows leaf
- 1 teaspoon dried oregano
- 1/2 teaspoon salt
- 1/4 teaspoon pepper
- 1 cup solidified corn, defrosted
- 1/4 cup minced crisp cilantro
- Discretionary garnishes: Cubed avocado, destroyed Monterey Jack cheddar

Guidelines:

In an enormous pan, heat quinoa and 2 cups water to the point of boiling. Decrease heat; spread and stew for 12-15 minutes or until water is retained. Expel from the warmth; lighten with a fork and put in a safe spot.

Then, in an enormous pan covered with cooking shower, cook the turkey, onion, red pepper and garlic over medium warmth until meat is never again pink and vegetables are delicate; channel. Mix in the bean stew powder, cumin and cinnamon; cook 2 minutes longer. Whenever wanted, present with discretionary garnishes.

Include the dark beans, tomatoes, zucchini, chipotle pepper, adobo sauce, sound leaf, oregano, salt, pepper and remaining water. Heat to the point of boiling. Diminish heat; spread and stew for 30 minutes. Mix in corn and quinoa; heat through. Dispose of narrows leaf; mix in cilantro. Present with discretionary fixings as wanted.

Freeze alternative: Freeze cooled stew in cooler compartments. To utilize, incompletely defrost in fridge medium-term. Warmth through in a pot, blending once in a while; include juices or water if vital.

Recipes For Wholesome Dinner

46.Chicken piccata with lemon sauce

INFGRIDENTS:

- 8 boneless skinless chicken bosom parts (4 ounces each)
- 1/2 cup egg substitute
- 2 tablespoons in addition to 1/4 cup dry white wine or chicken stock, isolated
- 5 tablespoons lemon juice, partitioned
- 3 garlic cloves, minced
- 1/8 teaspoon hot pepper sauce
- 1/2 cup generally useful flour
- 1/2 cup ground Parmesan cheddar
- 1/4 cup minced new parsley
- 1/2 teaspoon salt
- 3 teaspoons olive oil, partitioned
- 2 tablespoons spread
- Purchase Ingredients Asian noodle plate of mixed greens
- Sesame Ahi fish wraps with zesty nut sauce
- Chicken and green olives taquitos
- Protein power beans and green stuffed shells
- Mexican pizzas
- Curried cauliflower chickpea wraps
- Chicken parmesan meatballs
- Mexican Zucchini lasagna
- Fiery chicken pot stickers
- Spaghetti pasta with herbed mushroom cream sauce
- Sound quinoa make ahead goulash
- Veggie darling red curry with cooler tomato coconut sauce

Guidelines:

Straighten chicken to 1/4-in. thickness. In a shallow dish, join the egg substitute, 2 tablespoons wine, 2 tablespoons lemon juice, garlic and hot pepper sauce. In another shallow dish, consolidate the flour, Parmesan cheddar, parsley and salt. Coat chicken with flour blend, plunge in egg substitute blend, at that point cover again with flour blend.

In an enormous nonstick skillet, darker four chicken bosom parts in 1-1/2 teaspoons oil for 3-5 minutes on each side or until juices run clear. Evacuate and keep warm. Channel drippings. Rehash with staying chicken and oil. Expel and keep warm.

In a similar container, dissolve margarine. Include the rest of the wine and lemon juice. Heat to the point of boiling. Bubble, revealed, until sauce is diminished by a fourth. Shower over chicken.

47.Meatball taco bowls

INGRIDENTS:
Meatballs:

- 1 lb. Lean Ground Beef (sub any ground meat like pork, turkey or chicken)
- 1 Egg
- 1/4 cup finely cleaved Kale or crisp herbs like Parsley or Cilantro (discretionary)
- 1 tsp Salt
- 1/2 tsp Black Pepper
- Taco Bowls
- 2 cups Enchilada Sauce (we utilize custom made)
- 16 Meatballs (fixings recorded previously)
- 2 cups Cooked Rice, white or dark colored
- 1 Avocado, cut
- 1 cup locally acquired Salsa or Pico de Gallo
- 1 cup Shredded Cheese
- 1 Jalapeno, daintily cut (discretionary)
- 1 Tbsp Cilantro, cleaved
- 1 Lime, cut into wedges
- Tortilla Chips, for serving

Directions:
To Make/Freeze

In a huge bowl, join ground meat, eggs, kale (if utilizing), salt and pepper. Blend in with your hands just until equitably consolidated. Structure into 16 meatballs around 1-inch in distance across and place on a sheet dish fixed with foil.

In the event that utilizing inside several days, refrigerate for as long as 2 days.

In the event that freezing, place sheet container in cooler until meatballs are strong. Move to a cooler sack. Meatballs will keep in the cooler for 3 to 4 months.

To Cook

In a medium pot, bring enchilada sauce to a low stew. Include meatballs (no compelling reason to defrost first if meatballs were solidified). Stew meatballs until cooked through, 12 minutes assuming crisp and 20 minutes whenever solidified.

While meatballs stew, prep different fixings.

Amass taco bowls by garnish rice with meatballs and sauce, cut avocado, salsa, cheddar, jalapeño cuts, and cilantro. Present with lime wedges and tortilla chips.

48.Asian noodle salad

INGRIDENTS:

- 8 ounces in length slight entire wheat pasta noodles —, for example, spaghetti (use soba noodles to make gluten free)
- 24 ounces Mann's Broccoli Cole Slaw — 2 12-ounce sacks
- 4 ounces ground carrots
- 1/4 cup extra-virgin olive oil
- 1/4 cup rice vinegar
- 3 tablespoons nectar — utilize light agave nectar to make veggie lover
- 3 tablespoons smooth nutty spread
- 2 tablespoons low-sodium soy sauce — gluten free if necessary
- 1 tablespoon Sriracha pepper sauce — or garlic chile sauce, in addition to extra to taste
- 1 tablespoon minced new ginger
- 2 teaspoons minced garlic — around 4 cloves
- 3/4 cup broiled unsalted peanuts, — generally slashed
- 3/4 cup new cilantro — finely slashed

Directions:

Heat a huge pot of salted water to the point of boiling. Cook the noodles until still somewhat firm, as per bundle headings. Channel and flush quickly with cool water to evacuate the overabundance starch and stop the cooking, at that point move to a huge serving bowl. Include the broccoli cole slaw and carrots.

While the pasta cooks, whisk together the olive oil, rice vinegar, nectar, nutty spread, soy sauce, Sriarcha, ginger, and garlic. Pour over the noodle blend and hurl to consolidate. Include the peanuts and cilantro and hurl again. Serve chilled or at room temperature with extra Sriracha sauce as wanted.

Formula Notes

Asian Noodle Salad can be served cold or at room temperature. Store remains in the cooler in a water/air proof holder for as long as 3 days.

49.Sesame tuna wraps with spicy peanut sauce

INGREDIENTS:

For the lettuce wraps:

- 1-14-ounce Ahi fish filet
- 1/2 teaspoon toasted sesame oil
- 1/2 tablespoons highly contrasting sesame seeds
- salt and pepper to taste
- 12-16 leaves Boston bibb or Butter lettuce
- 1 mango, hollowed and cut slight
- 2 enormous carrots, stripped and cut into matchsticks
- 3 green onions, cut on a level plane
- 1/2 English cucumber, cut into matchsticks
- 1 avocado, cut meagerly
- 2-3 enormous leaves bok choy, cut slender vertically
- sesame seeds for decorate
- For the fiery nut sauce:
- 1/4 cup regular salted nutty spread, smooth
- 1/2-2 teaspoons fluid aminos, or soy sauce (contingent upon salt want)
- 1/2 teaspoon Srichacha
- 1/2 teaspoon garlic bean stew sauce
- 1 tablespoon unseasoned rice wine vinegar
- 1 teaspoon toasted sesame oil
- 2-2 1/2 tablespoons water
- 1 teaspoon nectar

Guidelines:

On an enormous serving platter or plate, place the lettuce leaves next to each other and uniformly disseminate the cut vegetables and mango among them.

On a little plate, brush all sides of the fish filet with the sesame oil and sprinkle with a smidgen of salt and crisp ground pepper. Press the sesame seeds onto each side and singe in a little skillet over medium high warmth for 1-2 minutes for every side (or until wanted doneness). Expel from warmth and let set for 5 minutes.

In the interim, in a little bowl, whisk together the sauce fixings until all around consolidated, including marginally more water if important. Taste en route for flavoring.

Daintily cut the fish along the grain and segment the pieces onto the readied lettuce leaves. Serve nearby the nut sauce. Appreciate!

50.Chicken with green olives tequitto

INGRIDENTS:

- 2 tablespoons additional virgin olive oil
- 3 to 4 pounds leg-thigh bits of chicken, cut in two, overabundance fat evacuated
- Salt and pepper to taste
- 1 huge onion, slashed
- 2 teaspoons stripped and minced ginger
- 1-inch cinnamon stick, or 1/4 teaspoon ground cinnamon
- 1 tablespoon minced garlic
- 1 teaspoon ground cumin
- 1 teaspoon paprika
- 2 cups chicken stock or water
- 1 ½ cups green olives, depleted and pitted
- Lemon juice to taste
- Hacked cilantro leaves for decorate

Guidelines:

Put oil in profound skillet or meal. Go warmth to medium-high and hold up a moment, until oil is hot. Include chicken, skin-side down, and dark colored it well, pivoting and turning pieces as vital and sprinkling with salt and pepper as they cook; 10 to 15 minutes all out. Go warmth to medium, evacuate chicken and pour off everything except 2 tablespoons of fat.

Include onion, ginger, cinnamon, garlic, cumin, paprika, 1/2 teaspoon or a greater amount of pepper and some salt and cook, blending periodically, for around 5 minutes, until onion mollifies. Add stock and raise warmth to medium-high; return chicken to dish, skin-side up. Cook at an exuberant stew for around 10 minutes. Add olives and keep on cooking until chicken is done, another 10 to 15 minutes or somewhere in the vicinity. Include lemon juice, at that point taste and alter flavoring. Trimming and serve.

51.Protein power beans and green stuffed shells

INGRIDENTS:

- Genuine or ocean salt
- Olive oil
- 12 oz. bundle kind sized shells (around 40)
- 1 lb. solidified cleaved spinach
- 2 to 3 cloves garlic, stripped and divided
- 15 to 16 oz. ricotta cheddar (ideally full fat/entire milk)
- 2 eggs
- 1 can white beans, (for example, cannellini), depleted and flushed
- ½ C green pesto, custom made or locally acquired
- Ground dark pepper
- 3 C (or more) marinara sauce
- Ground parmesan or pecorino cheddar (discretionary)

Guidelines:

Heat at any rate 5 quarts of water to the point of boiling in an enormous pot (or work in two littler clumps). Include a tablespoon of salt, a sprinkle of olive oil, and the shells. Bubble around 9 minutes (or until extremely still somewhat firm), blending sporadically to keep the shells isolated. Tenderly channel the shells in a colander, or scoop from the water with an opened spoon. Wash quickly with cool water. Line a rimmed heating sheet with cling wrap. At the point when the shells are sufficiently cool to deal with, separate them by hand, dumping out extra water and putting opening up in a solitary layer on the sheet container. Spread with progressively plastic wrap once practically cool.

Bring a couple of quarts of water (or utilize remaining pasta water, on the off chance that you didn't dump it out) to a bubble in a similar pot. Include solidified spinach and cook three minutes on high, until delicate. Line the colander with soggy paper towels on the off chance that the openings are enormous, at that point channel the spinach. Set colander over a bowl to deplete more while you start the filling.

Add only the garlic to a nourishment processor and run until it's finely hacked and adhering to the sides. Scratch down the sides of the bowl, at that point include the ricotta, eggs, beans, pesto, 1½ teaspoons salt, and a few toils of pepper (a major squeeze). Press the spinach in your grasp to deplete well of outstanding water, at that point add to different fixings in the nourishment processor. Run until practically smooth, with a couple of little bits of spinach still noticeable. I lean toward not to taste subsequent to including the crude egg, yet on the off chance that you think that its fundamental taste a little and modify flavoring to taste.

Preheat the broiler to 350 (F) and shower or gently oil a 9 x 13" skillet, in addition to another littler goulash dish (around 8 to 10 of the shells won't fit in the 9 x 13). To fill the shells, get each shell in turn, holding it open with thumb and pointer finger of your non-predominant hand. Scoop 3 to 4 tablespoons loading up with your other hand and scratch into the shell. The greater part of them won't look great, which is alright! Spot filled shells near one another in the readied container. Spoon sauce over the shells, leaving bits of the green filling unmistakable. Spread container with thwart and prepare for 30 minutes. Increment warmth to 375 (F), sprinkle shells with some ground parmesan (if utilizing), and heat revealed for another 5 to 10 minutes until cheddar is dissolved and abundance dampness is diminished. Cool 5 to 10 minutes, at that point serve alone or with a fresh plate of mixed greens as an afterthought!

52.Mexican pizza

INGRIDENTS:

- ground hamburger
- parcel of taco flavoring (or custom made)
- water
- oil
- corn tortillas
- refried beans
- red enchilada sauce
- destroyed cheddar
- roma tomato
- cut olives
- green onions

Guidelines:

Cook ground hamburger. Include taco flavoring and water and mix to consolidate.
Cook corn tortillas. Gently sauté them shortly of oil.

Collect. Spoon a slender layer of enchilada sauce over one corn tortilla, spread refried beans on and top with a spoonful of taco meat. Sprinkle cheddar over the meat and spot a second corn tortilla on top.

Top with enchilada sauce. Spread far layer of enchilada sauce over the tortilla and sprinkle with more cheddar.

Prepare at 400 degrees for around 10 minutes, until cheddar is liquefied and bubbly.

Trimming with olives, tomatoes, green onion and acrid cream. Slice into wedges to serve.

53.Curried cauliflower and chickpea wraps

INGREDIENTS:

- 1 Ginger Fresh
- 2 cloves Garlic
- 1 can Chickpeas
- 1 Red Onion
- 8 ounces Cauliflower Florets
- 1 teaspoon Garam Masala
- 2 tablespoons Arrowroot Starch
- 1 Lemon
- 1 pack Cilantro Fresh
- 1/4 cup Vegan Yogurt
- 4 Wraps
- 3 tablespoons Shredded Coconut
- 4 ounces Baby Spinach
- 1 tablespoon Vegetable Oil
- 1 teaspoon Salt and Pepper To taste

Directions:

Preheat the stove to 400 °F (205 °C). Strip and mince 1 tsp of the ginger. Mince the garlic. Channel and wash the chickpeas. Strip and meagerly cut the red onion. Split the lemon.

Coat a heating sheet with 1 tbsp vegetable oil. In an enormous bowl, consolidate the minced ginger, garlic, the juice from a large portion of the lemon, chickpeas, cut red onion, cauliflower florets, garam masala, arrowroot starch, and 1/2 tsp salt. Move to the preparing sheet and meal in the broiler until cauliflower is delicate and sautéed in places, around 20 to 25 minutes.

Hack the cilantro leaves and delicate stems. In a little bowl, whisk together the cilantro, yogurt, 1 tbsp lemon juice, and a spot of salt and pepper.

Spot the encloses by foil and pop them into the stove to warm around 3 to 4 minutes. Spot a little nonstick skillet over medium warmth and include the destroyed coconut. Toast, shaking the dish habitually until daintily cooked, around 2 to 3 minutes.

Gap the infant spinach and cooked vegetables between the warm wraps. Lay the cauliflower chickpea wraps on enormous plates and sprinkle with the cilantro sauce.Sprinkle with toasted coconut

54.Chicken parmesan meatballs

INGRIDENTS:

- 2 pounds ground chicken
- 3/4 cup panko breadcrumbs gluten free panko will work fine
- 1/4 cup finely minced onion
- 2 tablespoons minced parsley
- 2 cloves garlic minced
- get-up-and-go of 1 little lemon around 1 teaspoon
- 2 eggs
- 3/4 cup destroyed Pecorino Romano or Parmesan cheddar
- 1 teaspoon genuine salt
- 1/2 teaspoon crisply ground dark pepper
- 1 quart Five Minute Marinara Sauce
- 4-6 ounces mozzarella crisply cut

Directions:

Preheat the stove to 400 degrees, setting the rack in the upper third of the broiler. In a huge bowl, join everything aside from the marinara and the mozzarella. Softly combine, utilizing your hands or an enormous spoon. Scoop and shape into little meatballs and spot on a foil lined heating sheet. Spot the meatballs genuinely near one another on the plate to make them fit. Spoon about a half tablespoon of sauce over every meatball. Heat for 15 minutes.

Expel meatballs from the stove and increment the broiler temperature to cook. Spoon an extra half tablespoon of sauce over every meatball and top with a little square of mozzarella. (I cut the slight cuts into pieces around 1" square.) Broil an extra 3 minutes, until the cheddar has softened and turned brilliant. Present with extra sauce. Appreciate!

55.Mexican zucchini lasagna

INGRIDENTS:

- For the zoodles:
- 3-4 Large zucchinis * Read notes!
- 1 Tbsp Salt
- For the lasagna:
- 2 Tbsp Extra-virgin olive oil
- 1 lb Ground 99% without fat Turkey
- 1 Cup Onion diced (1 little onion)
- 1 Tbsp + 2 tsp Fresh garlic diced
- 1 Tbsp + 1 tsp Taco flavoring I generally make my own utilizing the formula connected!
- Pepper
- 3/4 Cup Tomato Sauce
- 3/4 Cup Salsa of decision
- 1 15 oz Container of light or without fat ricotta cheddar
- 1 Large egg
- 1/2 Cup Cilantro generally hacked + extra for embellish
- 8 oz Light Mexican mix cheddar ground (around 2 cups, immovably stuffed)
- 1 Large red pepper cleaved

Directions:

Preheat the stove to 350 degrees.

Utilizing a mandolin, cut the zucchini into slender cuts, around 1/8 inch thick, Spread them out level onto 2 treat sheets and sprinkle with 1 Tbsp salt (it's alright if some zoodles cover on the container)

Heat them for 15-20 minutes, until just delicately starting to dark colored, to get all the dampness out.

While the zoodles cook, heat the olive oil over medium/high warmth in the enormous container. Include the ground turkey, diced onion, diced garlic, taco flavoring, and a spot of pepper. Cook until the onion is delicate and the turkey is seared, around 10-12 minutes.

Once the zoodles are cooked, move them to a long bit of paper towel, spread with another bit of paper towel, and delicately press out as a lot of overabundance dampness as you can. Put in a safe spot.

In a medium bowl, mix together the tomato sauce and salsa.

In a different, medium bowl, utilize a fork to beat together the ricotta cheddar, egg and another touch of pepper. Put in a safe spot.

Splash a 9x13 inch heating dish with cooking shower.

Start by pouring a large portion of the sauce blend on the base, spreading out equally, trailed significantly the turkey. Layer a large portion of the zucchini noodles in a solitary layer, softly covering them, trailed considerably the ricotta blend. Tenderly spread out the ricotta to "seal in" in the zoodles.

Sprinkle a large portion of the cilantro over and afterward finish with a large portion of the ground Mexican mix cheddar.

Rehash the layers again, with the exception of include the slashed pepper top of the last layer of Mexican mix.

Turn the broiler up to 375 and spread the lasagna with tin foil.

Heat, secured, for 45 minutes. Reveal and heat an additional 10 minutes.

Turn the grill up to HIGH and sear for 2-3 minutes more, until the top is brilliant darker and bubbly!

Enhancement with additional cilantro (whenever wanted) and DEVOUR!

56.Fiery chicken pot stickers

INGRIDENTS:

- 1-pound ground chicken
- 1/2 cup destroyed cabbage
- 1 carrot, stripped and destroyed
- 2 cloves garlic, squeezed
- 2 green onions, meagerly cut
- 1 tablespoon diminished sodium soy sauce
- 1 tablespoon hoisin sauce
- 1 tablespoon naturally ground ginger
- 2 teaspoons sesame oil
- 1/4 teaspoon ground white pepper
- 36 won ton wrappers
- 2 tablespoons vegetable oil
- FOR THE HOT CHILI OIL SAUCE:
- 1/2 cup vegetable oil
- 1/4 cup dried red chillies, squashed
- 2 cloves garlic, minced

Guidelines:

Warmth vegetable oil in a little pan over medium warmth. Mix in squashed peppers and garlic, mixing every so often, until the oil arrives at 180 degrees F, around 8-10 minutes; put in a safe spot.

In an enormous bowl, join chicken, cabbage, carrot, garlic, green onions, soy sauce, hoisin sauce, ginger, sesame oil and white pepper.

To collect the dumplings, place wrappers on a work surface. Spoon 1 tablespoon of the chicken blend into the focal point of every wrapper. Utilizing your finger, rub the edges of the wrappers with water. Crease the mixture over the filling to make a half-moon shape, squeezing the edges to seal.

Warmth vegetable oil in a huge skillet over medium warmth. Include pot stickers in a solitary layer and cook until brilliant and fresh, around 2-3 minutes for each side. Serve promptly with hot stew oil sauce.

57.Spaghetti pasta with herbed mushroom sauce

INGREDIENTS:

- 200 grams/6.3 oz around a large portion of a pack of wheat slender spaghetti *
- 140 grams cleaned cleaved mushrooms 12-15 pieces*
- ¼ cup cream
- 3 cups milk
- 2 tablespoon cooking olive oil in addition to
- 2 teaspoon more oil or liquefied margarine to include mid-way
- 1.5 tablespoon flour
- ½ cup cleaved onions
- ¼ to ½ cup crisply ground parmesan cheddar
- Couple of bits of dark pepper
- Salt to taste
- 2 teaspoons dried or new thyme *
- Bunch of chiffonade new basil leaves

Directions:

Cook pasta still somewhat firm as indicated by the bundle.

While the pasta is cooking, we should begin making the sauce.

Warmth the 3 cups milk in the microwave for 3 minutes or on the stovetop until a stew.

At the same time heat 2 tablespoon oil in a non-stick container on medium high and cook the cleaved mushrooms. Cook for around 2 minutes.

From the outset the mushrooms will discharge some water, then it will evaporate in the long run and become fresh apiece.

Presently lessen the fire to medium include the onions and cook for 1 moment.

Presently include 2 teaspoons of softened spread and sprinkle some flour.

Mix for 20 seconds.

Include the warm milk mixing constantly to shape a smooth sauce.

When the sauce thicken i.e. goes to a stew, switch off the fire.

Presently include ¼ cup ground parmesan cheddar. Mix until smooth. For 30 seconds.

Presently include the salt, pepper and thyme.

Give a trial. Modify flavoring if necessary.

In interim pasta ought to be bubbled still somewhat firm.

Strain the warm water in a colander. Keep the tap running and pour cold water to stop it's cooking, channel all the water and hurl it with the sauce.

If not eating promptly, don't blend the pasta in the sauce. Keep the pasta separate, covered with oil and secured.

Serve warm with more sprinkle of parmesan cheddar. Appreciate!

58.Quinoa dish

INGRIDENTS:

- 1/2 cups quinoa, dry
- 2 tbsp avocado or coconut oil
- 2 garlic cloves, squashed
- 1/2 cups corn, canned or solidified
- 3 huge ringer peppers, hacked
- 1/2 medium jalapeño pepper, seeded and minced
- 1 tbsp cumin
- 15 oz container of dark beans, flushed and depleted
- 1 cup cilantro, finely hacked and partitioned
- 1/2 cup green onions, finely hacked and partitioned
- 2 cups Tex Mex cheddar, destroyed and separated
- 3/4 cup canned coconut milk
- 1/4 tsp salt

Directions:

Cook quinoa according to bundle directions and put in a safe spot. Preheat broiler to 350 F degrees.

Preheat huge clay non-stick skillet on medium warmth and twirl oil to cover.

Include garlic and cook for 30 seconds, mixing habitually. Include corn, chime peppers, jalapenos and cumin. Mix and sauté undisturbed for 3 minutes, mix again and sauté for an additional 3 minutes.

Move to a huge blending bowl alongside cooked quinoa, dark beans, 3/4 cup cilantro, 1/4 cup green onions, 1/2 cups cheddar, coconut milk and salt. Blend well, move to 8 x 11 preparing dish, sprinkle with staying 1/2 cup cheddar and heat for30 minutes revealed.

Expel from the broiler, sprinkle with staying 1/4 cup cilantro and 1/4 cup green onions. Serve warm

59.Red curry with tomato coconut sauce
INGRIDENTS:

- tablespoon lemon pizzazz (from 1 lemon) or 2 stalks lemongrass, slashed
- 1tablespoon cleaved shallot
- 2dried red bean stew pepper (chiles de arbol), seeded, toasted and doused for 20 minutes
- 3tablespoons minced garlic
- 2tablespoons ginger root, stripped and minced (around a 2-inch piece)
- 2teaspoons fish sauce
- 1tablespoon cumin seeds, toasted and ground
- 1tablespoon coriander seeds, toasted and ground
- 1teaspoon crisply ground white pepper

Guidelines:

Mesh the pizzazz from the lemon. Include the lemon pizzazz, shallot, chiles, garlic, ginger, fish sauce, cumin, coriander, white pepper, salt and 1/4 cup coconut milk to nourishment processor. Spread and procedure for 4 minutes or until the blend is smooth.

Mesh the pizzazz and crush the juice from the lime.

Warmth the oil in a 12-inch skillet over medium-high warmth. Include the shallot blend and cook for 2 minutes, mixing regularly.

Include the eggplant, remaining coconut milk, tofu, soup, lime pizzazz and cinnamon adhere to the skillet and warmth to a bubble. Lessen the warmth to medium-low. Cook for 10 minutes or until the eggplant is delicate, mixing every so often. Expel and dispose of the cinnamon stick. Mix in the lime juice and basil. Serve the eggplant blend with the rice.

60.Ground meat stroganoff

INGRIDENST:

- 1 lb lean ground meat
- 1 little onion diced
- 1 clove garlic minced
- 3/4 lb new mushrooms cut
- 3 tablespoons flour
- 2 cups meat stock
- salt and pepper to taste
- 2 teaspoons Worcestershire sauce
- 3/4 cup sharp cream
- 2 tablespoons new parsley

Directions:

Dark colored ground hamburger, onion and garlic (making an effort not to split it up something over the top) in a dish until no pink remains. Channel fat.

Include cut mushrooms and cook 2-3 minutes. Mix in flour and cook 1 progressively minute.

Include stock, Worcestershire sauce, salt and pepper and heat to the point of boiling. Lessen warmth and stew on low 10 minutes. Cook egg noodles as indicated by bundle headings.

Expel meat blend from the warmth, mix in sharp cream and parsley.

Serve over egg noodles.

61.Orzo with sundried tomatoes

INGREDIENTS:

- 1 lb boneless skinless chicken bosoms, diced into 3/4-inch pieces
- 1 Tbsp + 1 tsp olive oil
- Salt and crisply ground dark pepper
- 2 cloves garlic, minced
- 1/4 cups (8 oz) dry orzo pasta
- 2 3/4 cups low-sodium chicken stock, at that point more varying (don't utilize ordinary juices, it will be excessively salty)
- 1/3 cup sun dried tomato parts stuffed in oil with herbs (around 12 parts. Shake off a portion of the abundance oil), hacked fine in a nourishment processor
- 1/2 - 3/4 cup finely destroyed parmesan cheddar, to taste
- 1/3 cup cleaved crisp basil

Directions:

Warmth 1 Tbsp olive oil in a saute container over medium-high warmth.

Once gleaming include chicken, season gently with salt and pepper and cook until brilliant, around 3 minutes at that point pivot to inverse sides and cook until brilliant dark colored and cooked through, around 3 minutes. Move chicken to a plate, spread with foil to keep warm.

Include staying 1 tsp olive oil to saute dish at that point include garlic and saute 20 seconds, or just until daintily brilliant, at that point pour in chicken juices while scraping up cooked bits from base of skillet.

Heat stock to the point of boiling at that point include orzo pasta, lessen warmth to medium spread skillet with cover and permit to delicately bubble 5 minutes at that point reveal, mix and keep on bubbling revealed until orzo is delicate, around 5 minutes longer, blending at times (don't stress if there's still a little juices, it will give it some saucy-ness).

When pasta has cooked through hurl chicken in with orzo at that point expel from heat. Include parmesan cheddar and mix until dissolved, at that point hurl in sun dried tomatoes, basil and season with pepper (you shouldn't require any salt however include a little in the event that you'd think it needs it).

Add more juices to thin whenever wanted (as the pasta rests it will absorb abundance fluid and I enjoyed it with somewhat overabundance so I included somewhat more). Serve warm.

62.Cheesy stuffed chicken

INGRIDENTS:

- 2 scallions (meagerly cut)
- 2 seeded jalapeños (meagerly cut)
- 1/4 c. cilantro
- 1 tsp. lime pizzazz
- 4 oz. Monterey Jack cheddar (coarsely ground)
- 4 little boneless, skinless chicken bosoms
- 3 tbsp. olive oil
- Salt
- Pepper
- 3 tbsp. lime juice
- 2 ringer peppers (daintily cut)
- 1/2 little red onion (meagerly cut)
- 5 c. torn romaine lettuce

Guidelines:

Warmth broiler to 450°F. In bowl, consolidate scallions and seeded jalapeños, 1/4 cup cilantro (cleaved) and lime get-up-and-go, at that point hurl with Monterey Jack cheddar.

Supplement blade into thickest piece of every one of boneless, skinless chicken bosoms and move to and fro to make 2 1/2-inch pocket that is as wide as conceivable without experiencing. Stuff chicken with cheddar blend.

Warmth 2 tablespoons olive oil in enormous skillet on medium. Season chicken with salt and pepper and cook until brilliant darker on 1 side, 3 to 4 minutes. Turn chicken over and broil until cooked through, 10 to 12 minutes.

In the interim, in huge bowl, whisk together lime juice, 1 tablespoon olive oil and 1/2 teaspoon salt. Include ringer peppers and red onion and let sit 10 minutes, hurling sporadically. Hurl with romaine lettuce and 1 cup new cilantro. Present with chicken and lime wedges.

63.BAKED butternut squash rigatoni

INGRIDENTS:

- 1 enormous butternut squash
- 3 clove garlic
- 2 tbsp. olive oil
- 1 lb. rigatoni
- 1/2 c. substantial cream
- 3 c. destroyed fontina
- 2 tbsp. slashed crisp sage
- 1 tbsp. salt
- 1 tsp. naturally ground pepper
- 1 c. panko breadcrumbs

Guidelines:

Preheat broiler to 425 degrees F. In the meantime, in a huge bowl, hurl squash, garlic, and olive oil to cover. Spot on a huge, rimmed preparing sheet and dish until delicate, around 60 minutes. Move container to a wire rack and let cool marginally, around 10 minutes. Decrease stove to 350 degrees F.

In the meantime, heat a huge pot of salted water to the point of boiling and cook rigatoni as per bundle bearings. Channel and put in a safe spot.

Utilizing a blender or nourishment processor, purée held squash with overwhelming cream until smooth.

In a huge bowl, hurl squash puree withheld rigatoni, 2 cups fontina, savvy, salt, and pepper. Brush base and sides of a 9-by 13-inch preparing dish with olive oil. Move rigatoni-squash blend to dish.

In a little bowl, consolidate remaining fontina and panko. Sprinkle over pasta and heat until brilliant darker, 20 to 25 minutes.

www.ingramcontent.com/pod-product-compliance
Lightning Source LLC
Chambersburg PA
CBHW080629030426
42336CB00018B/3135